TRACE YOUR HAND BELOW!

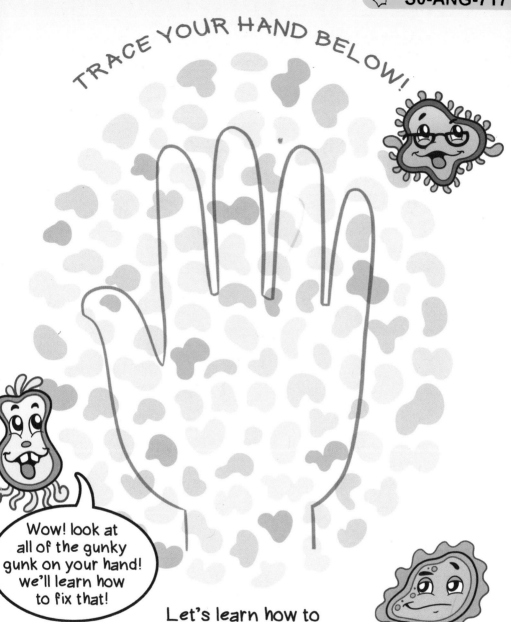

Wow! look at all of the gunky gunk on your hand! we'll learn how to fix that!

Let's learn how to wash away the gunk!

_____

Write your name here!

Fun Germ Facts!

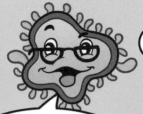

Yuck!

TWO TYPES OF GERMS

✸ VIRUS
The smallest type of germ. This is the kind that causes colds and the flu.

BACTERIA
A single cell germ. Many bacteria live in your body already and actually keep you healthy!

Did you know there are good and bad bacteria?

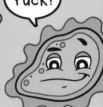

ATCHOOOO!

When you sneeze, germs can fly
3 - 5 feet
and travel up to
100 miles an hour!

Choo!

EUREKA!

In 1861, Louis Pasteur was the first to discover that people got sick because of germs!

!

HAND IT TO THE GERMS

There are usually millions of bacteria on each hand.

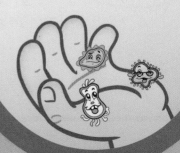

Wow! There are so many things to learn about germs!

Getting the Gunk off!

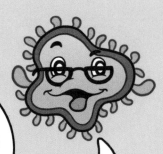

Hygiene is keeping both your body and your appearance neat and clean. This means washing your hands and brushing your teeth, as well as making sure to wear clean clothes and bathe regularly. Having good hygiene will keep you healthy and happy!

Washing your hands keeps germs from spreading so you and those around you don't get sick.

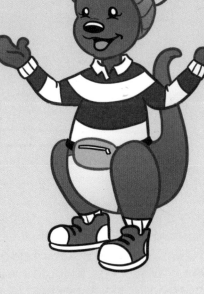

Brushing and flossing your teeth helps them grow healthy and strong.

Pewww!

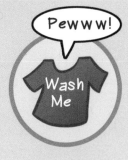

Wash Me

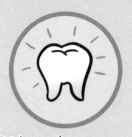

Did you know your teeth are alive? Caring for your CHOMPERS is important!

Bathing and wearing clean clothes helps you stay healthy and fresh so others want to be around you!

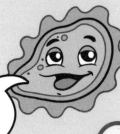

Gunk and the Tub

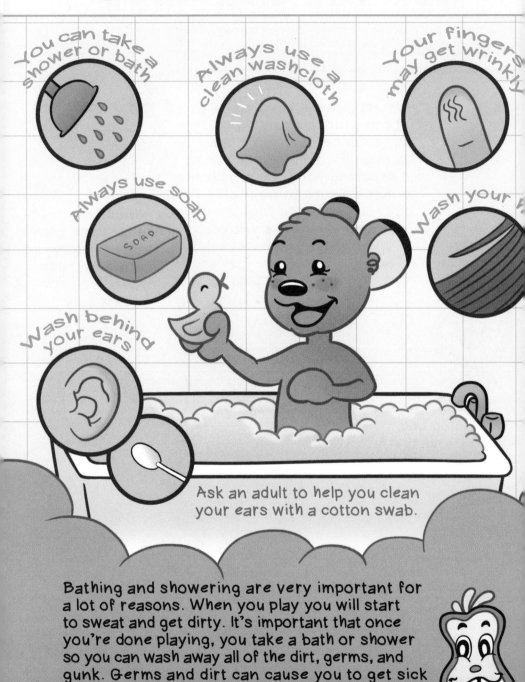

You can take a shower or bath

Always use a clean washcloth

Your fingers may get wrinkly

Always use soap

Wash your h...

Wash behind your ears

Ask an adult to help you clean your ears with a cotton swab.

Bathing and showering are very important for a lot of reasons. When you play you will start to sweat and get dirty. It's important that once you're done playing, you take a bath or shower so you can wash away all of the dirt, germs, and gunk. Germs and dirt can cause you to get sick and even start to hurt your skin if you go too long without bathing. Even if you don't feel like you're very sweaty or dirty, it's good to take a shower or bath before bedtime.

Don't Be a Gunk Mouth!

"Chew"se to care for your mouth!

Flossing is imporant to keep the spaces between your teeth clean and healthy.

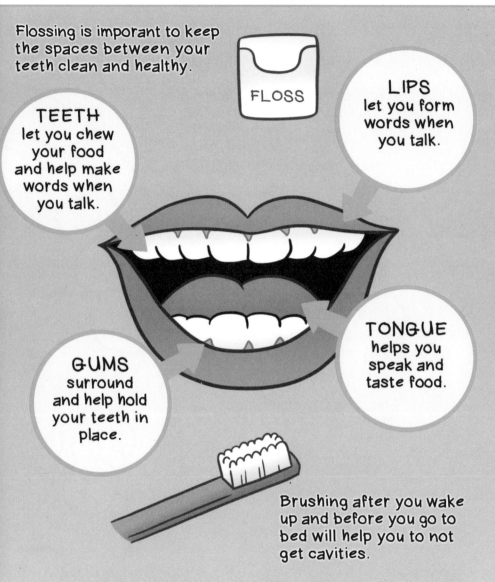

FLOSS

LIPS let you form words when you talk.

TEETH let you chew your food and help make words when you talk.

TONGUE helps you speak and taste food.

GUMS surround and help hold your teeth in place.

Brushing after you wake up and before you go to bed will help you to not get cavities.

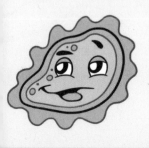

Every time you eat, food bits are left on and around your teeth. It's important to clean them so your smile stays healthy and strong. When brushing, keep going for 30 seconds or for a verse of your favorite song. Brush twice a day and floss once, because when you take care of your teeth, your teeth will take care of you! That's a lot to "chew" on!

All about Your Mouth!

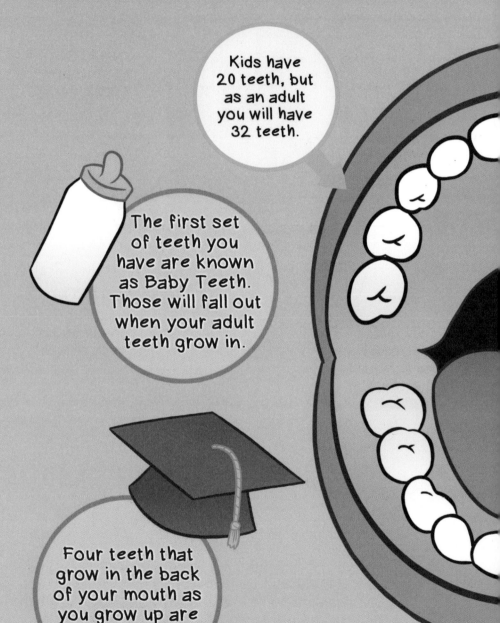

Kids have 20 teeth, but as an adult you will have 32 teeth.

The first set of teeth you have are known as Baby Teeth. Those will fall out when your adult teeth grow in.

Four teeth that grow in the back of your mouth as you grow up are called wisdom teeth.

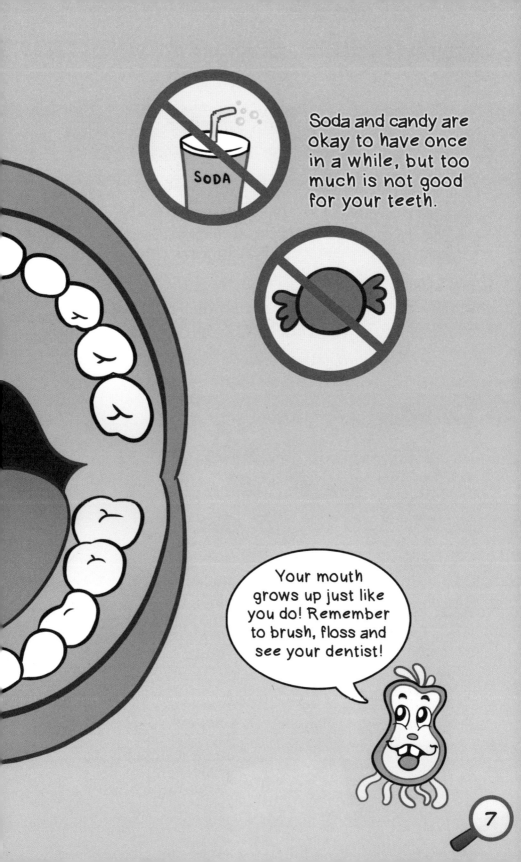

Soda and candy are okay to have once in a while, but too much is not good for your teeth.

Your mouth grows up just like you do! Remember to brush, floss and see your dentist!

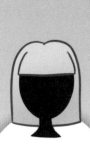

FINE HAIR
has thinner
strands

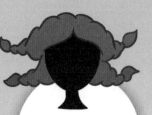

KINKY HAIR
is wiry and
curly

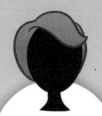

SHORT HAIR
means less to
deal with

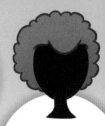

CURLY HAIR
is loopy and
thicker

TYPES of HAIR

Whatever type of hair you
have, it's important to keep
it neat and clean!

HAIR BRUSH

To keep your hair
tangle-free

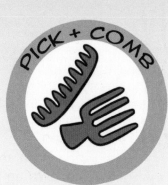

PICK + COMB

Also to keep
your hair
tangle-free

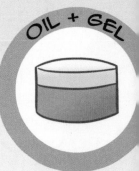

OIL + GEL

To keep your
hair moist and
in place

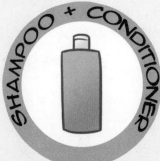

SHAMPOO + CONDITIONER

To clean and keep
your hair soft

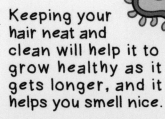

Keeping your
hair neat and
clean will help it to
grow healthy as it
gets longer, and it
helps you smell nice.

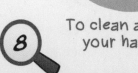

Finger Plan

Use each of your fingers to remember these tips when washing your hands!

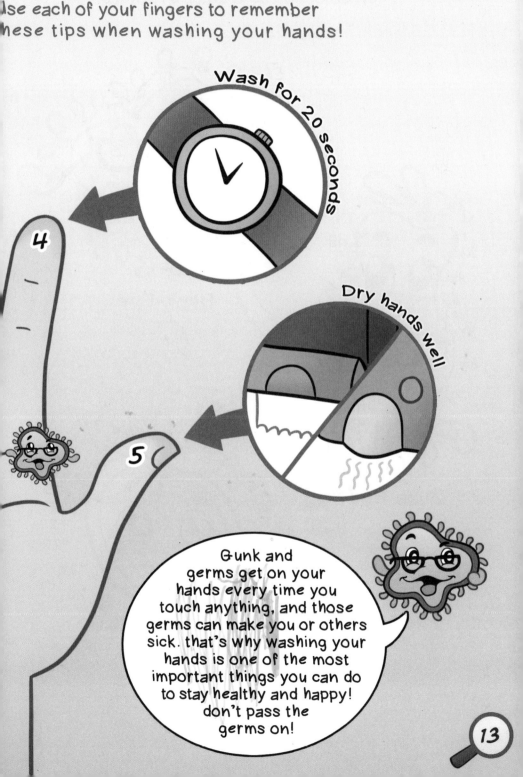

Wash for 20 seconds

Dry hands well

Gunk and germs get on your hands every time you touch anything, and those germs can make you or others sick. that's why washing your hands is one of the most important things you can do to stay healthy and happy! don't pass the germs on!

Connect the Dots

Then color in the Gunky Brothers!

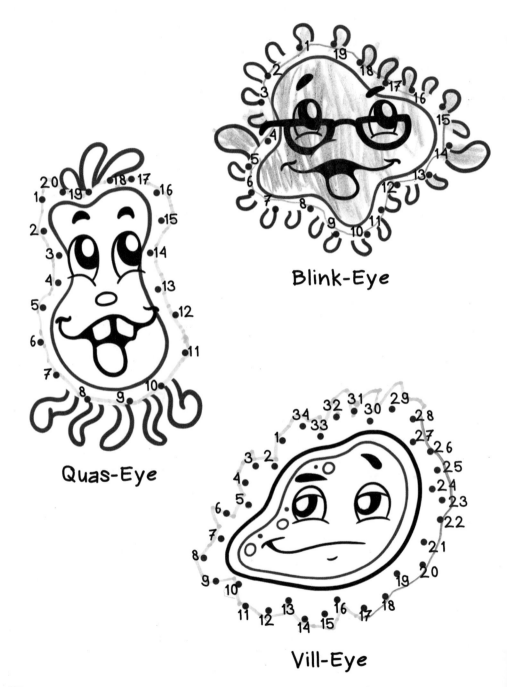

Blink-Eye

Quas-Eye

Vill-Eye

Find the Words

Fill in the blanks then find those
words in the puzzle below!

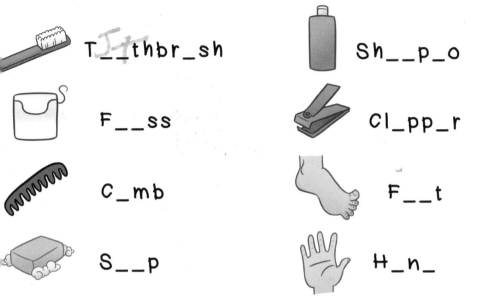

T__thbr_sh

Sh__p_o

F___ss

Cl_pp_r

C_mb

F___t

S__p

H_n_

```
F  L  O  S  S  L  B  T  H  J  F
A  X  L  M  O  R  Z  V  A  M  B
B  Q  R  P  A  M  X  D  N  Q  K
S  H  A  M  P  O  O  B  D  O  N
N  O  L  C  C  I  E  H  G  L  P
Z  T  O  O  T  H  B  R  U  S  H
T  F  R  M  C  L  I  P  P  E  R
V  U  S  B  X  P  N  F  O  O  T
```

15

Fill in the Answers

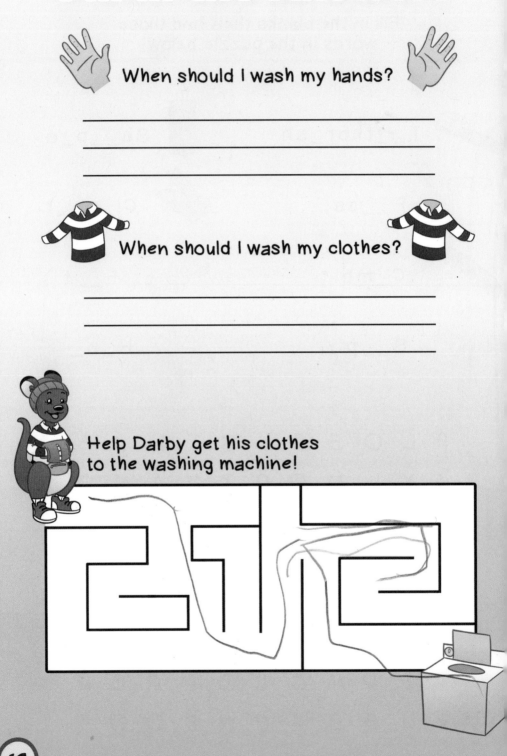

When should I wash my hands?

_____

_____

_____

When should I wash my clothes?

_____

_____

_____

Help Darby get his clothes
to the washing machine!

Read the words below and circle the pictures!

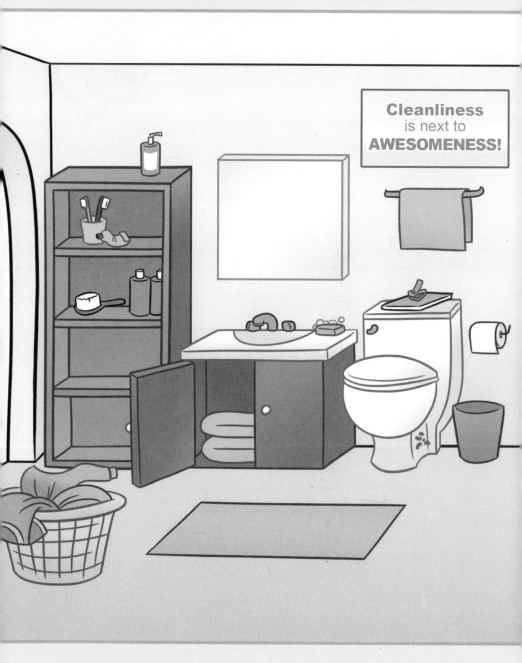

Cleanliness is next to AWESOMENESS!

Germs

Toothbrush

Soap

Hair Brush

Laundry Basket

Nail Clippers

Hand Sanitizer

Dry Towel

17

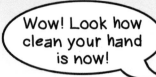

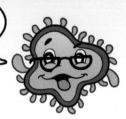

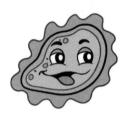

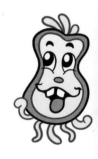

Trace your hand again!

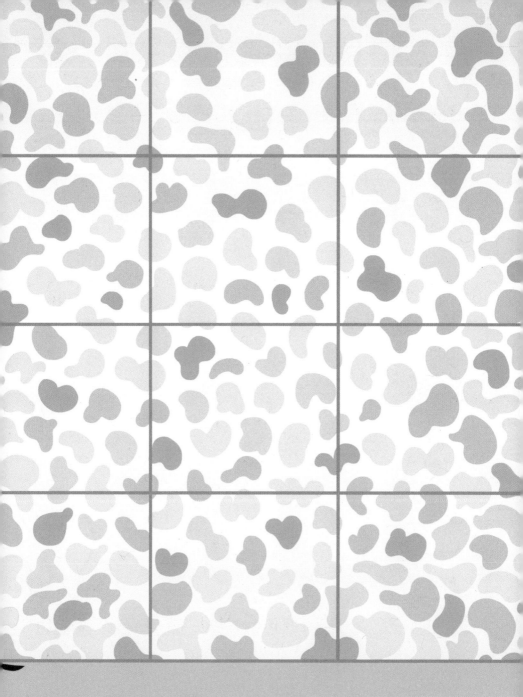

Have an adult help you cut out the puzzle pieces above. Then mix up the cards and lay them on a table with the germ pattern facing up. Turn over two cards at a time and try to match the cleaning tool with the part of the body you use it on.

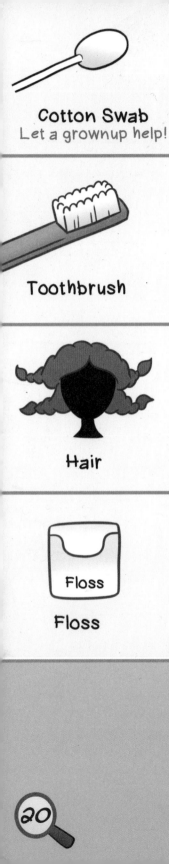

Cotton Swab
Let a grownup help!

Soap

Comb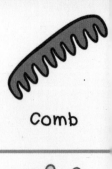

Toothbrush

Between Teeth

Hand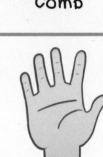

Hair

Ear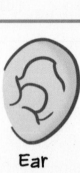

Clipper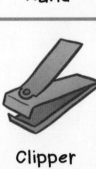

Floss

FingerNail

Tooth

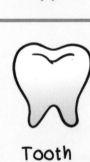

20